YOUR WAY, YOUR BEAUTIFUL HAIR BRAIDING

A Beginner's Handbook On Hair Braiding. Complete Guide On French Braids, Dutch Braids, Fishtail Braids And How To Keep Your Style Up-To-Date."

AURORA CELESTE

Table of Contents

CHAPTER ONE

INTRODUTION

Combining Style and Tradition

Braiding is an old way to style hair that has become a symbol of beauty, identity, and tradition that crosses time, culture, and location. This detailed guide will delve into the world of braiding, looking at where it came from, the different types of braids, and the necessary tools and supplies you'll need to make beautiful braided hairstyles. This trip through the art of braiding will help you figure out the secrets behind this time-honored skill, no matter how experienced you are.

HOW BRAID YOUR FIRST TIME

At its core, braiding is just weaving together several strands of hair to make a beautiful pattern. This style is useful because it keeps hair neat and easy to handle, but it can also be used in a lot of different ways. You can make braids simple or complicated, old-fashioned or modern, and you can change them to fit your style or the event.

What Braiding Means in Different Cultures

Braiding is a very important part of many cultures around the world. Hairstyles are more than just a way to style hair; they're also a way to tell stories, honor history, and show who you are.

African and African-American Traditions: Braids are a big part of identity and heritage in many African countries. Braids often show a person's age, social rank, and tribal affiliation by the complicated patterns and designs they have. For African Americans, braids have long been a strong sign of cultural pride and resistance.

Native American culture: In some Native American groups, braids have been used to show how important someone is in the tribe. Chiefs, fighters, and other respected people in the community wore different kinds of braids.

Asian Cultures: Braids are a popular part of traditional hairstyles in many Asian countries, such as India and China. The length and type of braids can show if someone is married or from a certain culture.

Viking and Celtic Traditions: In history, the Vikings and Celts were known for braiding their hair in very complicated ways that were often decorated with beads and jewellery. These complicated styles showed off their power and skill as warriors.

Modern Pop Culture: Braiding is still popular in today's world. Braids have become a sign of style and individuality, from the red carpet to the fashion shows.

DIFFERENT BRAID STYLES AND HOW THEY CAN BE USED

There are a lot of different types of braids, and each one has its own beauty and complexity. Whether you want an easy look for everyday life or a complicated masterpiece for a special event, there's a braid for you.

Straight Braid with Three Strands

A lot of braided haircuts start with the three-strand braid, which is also called the regular braid. It's easy and great for Beginners.

<u>***To braid three strands of hair***</u>

Split Your Hair Into Three Equal Parts

Cross the part on the right over the part in the middle.

Cross the part on the left over the part in the middle.

Hold it in place with a hair tie when you're done with these steps.

BRAID IN FRENCH

It starts at the crown and weaves hair from the top down. The French braid is a standard and classy style. It can be worn to a lot of different events, from relaxed to dressy. How to make a French braid:

Start with a small piece of hair at the head.

Split it up into three parts.

As you cross the strands over each other, add more hair from the sides bit by bit.

Hold your hair in place with a hair tie when you get to the nape of your neck.

BRAID IN DUTCH

The Dutch braid, which is also called a "inverted braid," looks like the French braid but makes the hair look raised and three-dimensional. It's great for giving your hair more depth.

How to make a Dutch braid

Like a French braid, start at the head.

Cross the strands under each other instead of over them.

Just like with the French braid, add more hair from the sides as you go.

Put a hair tie around the nape of your neck to keep it in place.

THE FISHTAIL BRAID

A trendy bohemian-style that looks complicated but is actually pretty easy to do is the fishtail braid. It is known for the way it is woven with two strands.

How to make a fishtail braid

Separate your hair into two equal parts.

Cut a small piece of yarn from the edge of the right piece and cross it over to connect it to the left piece.

Switch between sides and do this again and again until you reach the end.

Tie it off with a hair tie.

BRAID WITH WATERFALL

The waterfall braid makes it look like the strands are falling like a waterfall. It has a sweet and fun look.

How to make a waterfall braid

Begin with a small area of hair near your head.

Split it up into three parts.

Drop the bottom strand and pick up a new piece of hair from the top as you braid.

Keep doing this until you get the waterfall effect.

Tie it off with a hair tie.

CORNROWS WITH BOXER BRAIDS

Cross-over braids, or boxer braids, are close to the head and tight. They can be simple or complex. People with wavy or curly hair often wear them as a protective style.

How to make boxer braids

Split your hair into little chunks.

Start braiding at the bottom of your hair and add more hair to each part as you go.

Keep tying your hair tightly against your head.

Use hair ties to hold the ends together.

THE MOST IMPORTANT TOOLS AND SUPPLIES FOR BRAIDING

It is very important to have the right tools and supplies on hand before you start braiding. Not only will these things make the process easy, they will also make sure that your braids look great.

1. Hairbrush or Comb: Before you start braiding, a good hairbrush or comb can help you get rid of knots and smooth out your hair.

2. Hair Ties: You need hair ties or elastics to keep the ends of your knots in place. For less damage, choose hair ties that don't snag or are covered in cloth.

3. You can use hairpins or Bobby pins to hold down loose ends or tuck away extra strands while you braid.

4. Spray or Gel for Hair: Spray or gel for hair helps keep frizz and flyaways in check, so your braids stay in place.

5. Hair Oil or Serum: Putting on a light hair oil or serum before braiding can give your hair shine and keep it from drying out.

6. Hair Extensions (Optional): You can use hair extensions to get the look you want if you want to make your braids longer or fuller.

7. Any extras you want: You can add beads, ribbons, and other hair items to your braids to make them more personal and unique.

8. Mirror: You need a handheld or wall-mounted mirror so you can see how your braids are coming along from different directions.

There are a lot of different ways to braid your hair, whether you're getting ready for a special event, showing off your cultural background, or just looking for a new look. So, get your tools together and get some ideas. Then let's start this creative trip through braiding.

CHAPTER TWO

HOW TO GET YOUR HAIR READY FOR BRAIDING

The Basics for Making Beautiful Braids

It's important to prepare your hair properly before you start making beautiful braided hairstyles. Cleaning and conditioning your hair makes it easy to braid. This will make sure that your braids look great and stay in place. This part will talk about how important it is to keep your hair clean and moisturized. It will also give you tips on how to shampoo and condition your hair properly, and it will look at how different hair types can affect the braiding process.

Why clean, well-moisturized hair is important

1. Hair that is clean

Cleaning your hair is important for braiding for a number of reasons:

Better Control: Hair that is clean is easier to style and work with, which makes braiding go more smoothly and quickly.

Better Absorption of Products: Shampooing gets rid of oil and product buildup on your head and hair, which makes it easier for any styling or moisturising products you use afterward to work.

Less Frizz: Hair that is clean is less likely to have flyaways and frizz, which makes knots look neater and more polished.

Longer-Lasting Braids: Braids tend to stay in place better when hair is clean, since there aren't any oils or dirt left behind that could make them slip or come apart.

2. Hair that's well-hydrated

Keeping your hair moisturized is important for its health and look. This is especially true before braiding, since braids can sometimes make hair dry.

Some benefits of hair that is well moisturized are:

Less Breakage: Hair that is moisturized is less likely to break, so your hair stays healthy and strong while you braid it and afterward.

Because hair that has been moisturized is more flexible, it is easier to braid without damaging or stressing the strands.

The right amount of moisture gives hair a healthy sheen that can make your braided styles look even better.

HOW TO SHAMPOO YOUR HAIR

1. How to Pick the Best Shampoo

The first step in properly preparing your hair is to choose the right shampoo for your hair type. There are different soaps for different needs, such as

Clarifying shampoo is great for getting rid of a lot of product buildup.

Shampoo that moisturizes hair is great for hair that is dry or stressed and needs extra moisture.

Shampoo without sulphates is good for people with sensitive scalps or dyed hair.

2. How to Shampoo Correctly

Follow these steps to get the most out of your shampoo:

Wet Your Hair: First, use warm water to fully wet your hair. This helps the surface of the hair open up, which makes it easier for the shampoo to clean.

Use the Right Amount: Put a little shampoo on your palm—about the size of a quarter—and rub it in. The amount can be changed based on the length and thickness of your hair.

Massage Carefully: Use your fingertips, not your nails, to rub the shampoo into your hair. Cleanse the head and roots to get rid of buildup, dirt, and oils.

Rinse Well: Use cold water to rinse your hair until all the shampoo is gone. Make sure there is no residue left behind, as this can make your hair feel heavy or greasy.

HOW TO CHOOSE THE RIGHT CONDITIONER

After washing, you need to condition your hair to bring back the moisture. Pick a conditioner that goes well with your shampoo and hair type:

Standard Conditioner is good for most hair types and gives hair basic wetness.

Deep conditioners are great for hair that is dry or damaged because they deeply moisturize and fix the hair.

Leave-In Conditioner is a light choice that can be used every day to keep hair moist and free of tangles.

How to Use Conditioner Correctly

When you put conditioner on your hair, remember these tips:

Focus on the Ends: The mid-lengths and ends of your hair are more likely to be dry and damaged, so put most of the conditioner there.

Don't Put Conditioner On Your Scalp: Putting conditioner on your scalp can make your hair look oily.

Use a Wide-Tooth Comb: Once you're done conditioning your hair, use a wide-tooth comb to spread it out evenly and get rid of any knots.

<u>***Rinsing out conditioner***</u>

Time: Leave the conditioner in your hair for as long as the directions say to (usually one to two minutes) so it can moisturise and work its magic.

Rinse Well: Use cool water to rinse your hair well to seal the cuticle and keep the moisture in. Make sure there is no residue left over.

LEARNING ABOUT THE DIFFERENT TYPES OF HAIR

When getting ready to braid, different types of hair need different care and attention. To give you an idea of how different hair types might affect the braiding process, here they are:

1. Hair that is straight

Getting ready: Straight hair is usually easy to work with and might not need as much moisture as other hair types. But it's very important to make sure your hair is clean and free of extra oil.

When braiding, straight hair can hold knots well, but you need to use the right products to keep them from slipping.

2. Curly Hair

To keep your hair's natural structure, you should use a mix of moisturizing and light products when getting ready.

Braiding: Soft, romantic knots that hold their shape well can be made with wavy hair.

3. Hair Curls

To get ready, deep treatment is very important for curly hair because it tends to be dry. Carefully untangle your hair so that it doesn't break.

Braiding: Curly hair can make braids that are full and have lots of different textures. The natural feel can help the braids stay put.

4. Hair that is curly orkinky

Get ready: Hair that is curly or wavy needs to be thoroughly moisturized and detangled. Leave-in cleansers and oils might be a good idea.

Braiding: These hair types can be braided into beautiful, complex styles that have their own feel.

To get beautiful braided hairstyles that last, you need to make sure your hair is properly prepped. Keeping your hair clean and moisturized not only makes your braids look better, but it also helps your hair stay healthy in general. You can braid your hair successfully if you know what kind of hair you have and use the right shampoo and conditioner on it. The chapters that follow will go into detail about different braiding styles and techniques, giving you the chance to discover all the different ways this ancient art form can be used.

CHAPTER THREE

HOW TO DO BASIC BRAIDING

How to Do the Three-Strand Braid

The three-strand braid, which is also called the "regular braid," is the base for many braided hairstyles. It's a classic style that will never go out of style and can be used for a wide range of occasions, from everyday looks to fancy updos. This complete guide will teach you how to make a three-strand braid by giving you step-by-step instructions, answering common questions, and giving you useful tips that will help you get a perfect braid every time.

How to Understand the Three-Strand Braid

What does a three-strand braid look like?

A three-strand braid is a simple but beautiful way to braid hair. It is made by weaving three sections of hair over and under each other to make a pattern. The most basic way to braid, and it's what more complicated braid styles are built on. To learn how to do other types of braiding, you must first learn how to make a neat and even three-strand braid.

What kind of hair can be used for a three-strand braid?

• You can braid three strands of hair like this, even if your hair is straight, wavy, curly, or coily. But as we've talked about in earlier chapters, it's important to make sure your hair is clean, moisturised, and free of tangles before you braid it.

What length of hair do I need for a three-strand braid?

• You can braid three strands of hair that is any length, from short to long. Longer hair, on the other hand, lets you make braids that are more complicated and unique.

Can I braid my hair into a three-strand braid without help?

• Yes, a three-strand braid is one of the simplest braiding techniques and can be done on your hair without help. With practice, you'll become more skilled at tying your hair neatly and evenly.

How do I make my three-strand braid look even and tight?

• We'll address this question in detail in the tips part below, so keep reading for valuable advice on achieving a perfect braid.

STEP-BY-STEP INSTRUCTIONS FOR CREATING A THREE-STRAND BRAID

Tools and Products You'll Need:

- *Comb or hairbrush*

- *Hair tie (elastic band)*

- *Mirror (optional, for better vision)*

Step 1: Prepare Your Hair

1.Detangle Your Hair: Start with clean, detangled hair. Use a comb or hairbrush to remove any knots or tangles. This step is important for achieving a smooth braid. Decide where you want your braid to start. You can create a center part or a side part, based on your preferred style. Start with a centre part for a basic look.

Step 2: Split your hair into three parts.

1.Take a small piece of hair from the top of your head, close to where you part it, and split it into three equal strands. These are the three parts of your knot.

Step 3: Start braiding.

1.Cross the Right Strand Over the Middle Strand: With your right thumb and fingers, hold the right strand. It will become the new middle strand when you cross it over the middle strand.

2.Cross the Left Strand Over the New Middle Strand: With your left thumb and fingers, hold the left strand. Cross it over the new middle strand, which in the last step was the right strand. The new middle strand is now it.

3.Do it again: Keep switching between crossing the left strand over the middle strand and crossing the right strand over the middle strand. This process of weaving makes the braid.

Step 4: Tie the braid in place.

1.Continue Braiding: Weave your hair again and again until you reach the end. To make a regular braid, try to keep the tension the same on all of the strands.

2.Put a hair tie around the end of the braid to keep it in place. Once you've braided your hair to the length you want, do this. Make sure it fits well, but not too well, so you don't feel uncomfortable.

Step 5: Add the finishing touches

1.Change the Braid: To make the braid a little less tight, gently pull on the sides of it. In this way, the braid looks thicker and less tight.

2.Optional: For an easy look, you can leave the braid alone, or you can try out different ways to style it. You could, for instance, wrap the braid around your head to make a crown braid or put it up to wear it up.

ADVICE ON HOW TO KEEP THE BRAID TENSE AND EVEN

It takes skill and close attention to detail to make a three-strand braid that is neatly woven and even. To help you make a pretty braid, here are some tips:

1. Keep Strand Sizes Consistent:

- Make sure that each of the three strands you split your hair into at the start is about the same size. This helps make a braid that is balanced.

2. Controlling your tension

- Make sure that the tension on each strand stays the same as you weave. Do not pull on one strand too tightly, as this can change the shape of the braid.

3. Keep the Strands neat

- Comb or brush each strand before sewing to keep the braid from getting tangled or having uneven spots.

4. Mirrors can help you see better

- If you're braiding your hair in the back, look at yourself in the mirror or ask someone to help you keep the tightness even and the line straight.

5. It's important to practise

• Like any other skill, braiding gets better with practice. If your first few tries aren't perfect, don't give up. Just keep training, and you'll get better.

6. Try out a number of different styles

• Once you know how to do the basic three-strand braid, try the French braid, the Dutch braid, the fishtail braid, and other versions to get better at braiding.

Three-strand braids are the most basic type of braiding and can be used as a base for many different hairstyles. You can make beautiful braids that are perfect for any event by following the step-by-step steps and using the tips for keeping the tension and evenness. When you feel more comfortable with your braiding skills, you'll be ready to try out more complicated braid styles.

French, Dutch, and fishtail braids are intermediate braids that can take your hairstyle to the next level.

There are as many options when it comes to braiding as there are styles. As you get better at braiding, you'll find more complex and interesting ways to do it than just the basic three-strand braid. The French braid, the Dutch braid, and the fishtail braid are all intermediate braids that we'll talk about in this complete guide. We'll give you detailed, step-by-step steps on how to make each style, look at different versions for different events, and give you troubleshooting tips to fix common problems.

HOW TO BEND BRAIDS IN THE MIDDLE

1. Braid in French

The French braid is a classic and classy hairstyle that gives your hair depth and style. It's a braid that can be worn with or without makeup, for everyday or formal events.

HOW TO DO A FRENCH BRAID, STEP BY STEP

1.Get your hair ready. Begin by making sure it is clean and wet. First, brush your hair to get rid of any knots. Then, choose where you want the braid to start.

2.Your Hair: Split a piece of hair at the crown of your head into three equal strands. Hold them like you would a normal braid with three strands.

3.For the first step of the braid, cross the right strand over the middle strand, just like you would.

4.Add Hair: From the right side of your head, pull out a small piece of hair and weave it into the right strand as you cross it over the middle.

5.Cross the left strand over the middle strand and add a small piece of hair from the left side of your head to the left strand. Do this again on the left side.

6.To keep braiding, do steps 4 and 5 again, switching sides each time, and keep braiding your hair down. Remember to add hair from both sides every time you cross your hair over.

7.Once you've braided all the way down, keep going with a normal three-strand braid until you hit the end of your hair. Tie it off with a hair tie.

VARIOUS FORMS

• French Braid crown: Make a French braid that looks like a crown and wrap it around your head.

• Double French Braid: For a trendy look, split your hair in half and do a French braid on each side.

2. Braid in Dutch

The Dutch braid, which is also called a reversed braid, gives hair a unique 3D look. It's a great choice for making haircuts that stand out.

HOW TO DO A DUTCH BRAID, STEP BY STEP

1.Get your hair ready. Begin by making sure it is clean and wet. Brush your hair to get rid of knots.

2.Split Your Hair: Just like you would for a regular braid, split a piece of hair at the top of your head into three equal strands.

3.To start the braid, cross the right strand under the middle strand instead of over it.

4.Add Hair: Grab a small piece of hair from the right side of your head and add it to the right strand as you cross it under the middle.

5.Cross the left strand under the middle strand and add a small piece of hair from the left side of your head to the left strand. Do this again on the left side.

6.To keep braiding, do steps 4 and 5 again, switching sides each time, and keep braiding your hair down. For each crossing, make sure you add hair from both sides.

7.Once you've braided all the way down, keep going with a normal three-strand braid until you hit the end of your hair. Tie it off with a hair tie.

VARIOUS FORMS

You can make a Dutch braid cap that goes around your head like a crown.

This is a bold and trendy way to wear your hair. Split your hair into two parts and make Dutch braids on each side.

The fishtail braid

The fishtail braid gives off a cool and free spirit vibe. It looks hard to make at first, but it's actually very easy once you get the hang of it.

HOW TO MAKE A FISHTAIL BRAID, STEP BY STEP

1.Get your hair ready. Begin by making sure it is clean and wet. Brush your hair to get rid of knots.

2.Split Your Hair: Put all of your hair into one ball. Split it into two equal parts.

3.Hold one piece in each hand to start the braid. Bring a short piece of hair from the edge of the right section to the left section and cross it over.

4.Do it again on the left side: take a short piece of hair from the left side's edge and cross it over to the right side.

5.Keep Braiding: To keep braiding your hair down, keep going through steps 3 and 4, switching sides each time. When you cross over, make sure to take a few small pieces.

6.Protect the Braid: Use a hair tie to hold the end of the braid in place when you're done braiding all the way down.

VARIOUS FORMS

This is a messy fishtail braid. To make it look casual, pull the strands apart and loosen them up.

• Side Fishtail Braid: For a stylish, uneven look, place a fishtail braid on one side of your head.

HOW TO FIX PROBLEMS WITH INTERMEDIATE BRAIDS

It can be hard to do intermediate braids, but you can get through them with experience and the right techniques:

1. Strands That Slip: • Solution: With each crossing, make sure to add hair from both sides in the same way. This will help keep the braid together so that the pieces don't fall out.

2. Uneven Stress: • Solution: Work on keeping the tightness the same on both sides of the braid. To make sure the braid is even, gently tug on the sides as you go.

3. Scalp Tight: • If braiding makes your head feel too tight or painful, loosen the braid a bit by gently pulling on the sides.

4. Too Much Loose Braid: When adding hair to your braid, make sure you take small pieces so that it doesn't feel too loose. This will make the weave tighter.

5. Lack of Evenness: To fix this, use a mirror to look at the braid from different directions while you work. To get a finished look, fix any parts that aren't level.

The French braid, the Dutch braid, and the fishtail braid are all intermediate braids that can be styled in a lot of different ways. You can change these braids to fit different events and your own tastes. With this guide's step-by-step steps, different variations, and troubleshooting tips, you'll be able to master these beautiful braiding styles. As you practice and try out different styles, you will get better at braiding, and you will be able to easily make complicated and beautiful hairstyles.

CHAPTER FOUR

MORE ADVANCED BRAIDING STYLES

How to Do Waterfall, Rope, and Crown Braids

Your trip through the world of braiding will continue as you learn more advanced techniques that let you make beautiful and complicated hairstyles. The waterfall braid, the rope braid, and the crown braid are the three advanced braiding styles we'll talk about in this complete guide. We'll show you how to do these complicated styles step by step and give you helpful tips along the way. We'll also tell you when and where to wear them based on your own tastes and the situation.

GETTING BETTER AT BRAIDING

1. Braid with Waterfall

The waterfall braid is a cute and sweet style that makes it look like the hair is falling like a waterfall. You can add a bit of elegance to your look with this.

Details on how to do a waterfall braid, including what you'll need and how to do it.

A comb or a hairbrush

Hair tie with a stretchy band

Mirror (not required, but can help you see better)

Get your hair ready: Begin by making sure your hair is clean and wet. Brush your hair to get rid of knots.

Split your hair in half and choose where to start the waterfall braid. Most of the time, it starts near the temple in the front of your head. Cut a small piece of hair into three equal strands.

Start the Braid: Begin braiding like you would for a normal three-strand braid. First cross the right strand over the middle. Then, cross the left strand over the middle strand that you just made.

Add Hair: After the first two crossing steps, release the right strand and let it hang loose. Take a new piece of hair from the top of your head and put it just behind where you started the braid. This is now the right strand.

Repeat: Keep braiding. Every time you cross the right strand over the middle strand, add a new piece of hair from the top of your head to it. Leave the left thread hanging down.

If you want the braid to be a certain length or go to the other side of your head, tie off the end of it with a hair tie.

HOW TO DO WATERFALL BRAIDS

To keep the look even and balanced, make sure that the pieces of hair you pull out and put back in are all about the same thickness.

To make a smooth waterfall effect, work on your hand moves and coordination.

Braid a rope

You can also call this style a twist or rope braid. It gives your hair a unique and textured look. This look is very flexible and can be dressed up or down depending on the event.

What You'll Need to Make a Rope Braid: Step-by-Step Instructions

A comb or a hairbrush

Hair tie with a stretchy band

Mirror (not required, but can help you see better)

Get your hair ready: Begin by making sure your hair is clean and wet. Brush your hair to get rid of knots.

Separate Your Hair: Separate your hair into two equal parts.

Start the braid: Take one piece in each hand. Turn each part to the right (clockwise) one at a time.

Wrap It Up: Once you've turned each piece around, grab both of them and twist them together to the left (anticlockwise).

Hold the Braid in Place: Use a hair tie to hold the braid in place once you've turned all the way down to the ends.

When making a rope braid, make sure to twist each part tightly before joining them. This will make the braid look neat and clear.

You can make a rope braid on one side of your head and then use it in other braided ways for a more complex look.

Braid the crown

The crown braid, which is also called a halo braid or milkmaid braid, is a royal and classy style that goes around your head like a crown. It's great for formal events and special situations.

What You'll Need to Make a Crown Braid:

Step-by-Step Instructions

A comb or a hairbrush

Hair tie with a stretchy band

Pins for hair

Get your hair ready: Begin by making sure your hair is clean and wet. Brush your hair to get rid of knots.

Make a Centre Part: Make a centre part in your hair to split it into two equal parts, like you're putting together pigtails.

Start the braid on one side

Making a regular three-strand braid starts with one part. Cross the right strand over the middle strand and then the left strand over the new middle strand.

Make this braid go all the way down your hair, and then use a hair tie to hold the end in place.

Do it again on the other side

Follow the same steps make another three-strand braid on the other piece of hair.

Wrap the braids up

Place the beginning of the crown braid on one of the braids that you've brought up and over your head.

Use bobby pins to hold the end of this braid in place, then tuck it under the other braid to hide it.

Do the same thing with the other braid. Place it where the first braid ended and use bobby pins to hold it in place.

Make changes and lock

As needed, use bobby pins to keep any free parts in place and the braids from moving.

Finish off the look

You can use bobby pins to hold the ends of the braids under the crown braid for a smooth look.

Crown Braid Tips

To make braids that are even and balanced, practise the skill on both sides.

Move the braids around to get the crown shape you want, and then use bobby pins to keep them in place.

How to Wear These Braids and When

Each of these advanced braided styles gives you a different look that you can wear to different events and places:

The waterfall braid is great for weddings, romantic dates, or any other time you want to look elegant and fun with your hair.

Rope Braid: Can be worn to both relaxed and dressy events. You can wear it with casual clothes or dressier ones to add texture and drama.

Crown braid: This style looks great at weddings, proms, and other formal events. It gives off an air of royal grace and is perfect for important events.

You can get better at braiding by learning more advanced styles like the waterfall braid, rope braid, and crown braid. These styles let you make more complicated and beautiful haircuts. You can learn these advanced techniques and change them to fit different situations and your own tastes by following the step-by-step steps and tips in this guide. These advanced braiding styles let you explore and show off your creativity in a lot of different ways. You can go for a romantic and playful look, a style with lots of different textures, or an elegant and royal crown braid.

CHAPTER FIVE

HOW TO KEEP YOUR STYLE UP-TO-DATE AND YOUR HAIR HEALTHY

Braided haircuts are stylish, versatile, and can add a little something extra to your look. But, like any other haircut, they need to be taken care of properly to stay beautiful and keep your hair healthy. This complete guide will go over all the important things you need to know to take care of braided hair, from washing and cleaning to taking the braids out safely and keeping your hair safe while you sleep and do physical activities. Following these tips will help you avoid damage, make your braids last longer, and keep your hair healthy and bright.

The Basics

When you take care of your braided hair, you're not only keeping the style, but also your natural hair healthy. Simple care tips are given below:

1. Cleanse your scalp

• Cleanse your scalp: Use a scalp wash or dry shampoo to get rid of buildup and extra oil while your braids are in. Put it on your head directly and gently rub it in. This keeps you feeling fresh and cuts down on itching.

When you wash your hair normally, you can still do it with braids. Don't use too much of a sulfate-free shampoo, and just focus on the head. Rinse your hair well, but don't rub or manipulate it too much to keep it from frizzing.

2. Staying hydrated is important

• Use a leave-in conditioner. Put a leave-in conditioner on your braids and head to keep your natural hair moist. This keeps the hair from getting dry and breaking.

• Put oil on your scalp: Apply a light hair oil to your head every once in a while to keep it moist. With a dropper, you can apply the oil straight to your scalp without getting it all over your braids.

3. Don't overstyle

• Don't manipulate your braids too much: try to limit how often you touch, twist, or pull on them. Too much twisting can make hair frizzy and break.

• Protective Styles: If you want to change your look, don't fix your braids often. Instead, choose protective styles that are easy to change, like buns or updos.

4. Care at Night

• Silk or Satin cover: Sleeping on a silk or satin cover keeps your braids from getting frizzy by reducing friction. Before going to bed, you can also put a silk or satin scarf around your hair.

• Tie Braids Loosely: If your braids are long, tie them loosely with a scrunchie or a cloth hair tie before bed to keep them from getting tangled.

HOW TO WASH AND CONDITION BRAIDED HAIR

Keeping your hair clean and moisturized is important for both the health of your natural hair underneath the braids and the life of the braids.

HOW TO WASH BRAIDED HAIR

1. Water Down Shampoo: In a spray bottle, mix a mild, sulfate-free shampoo with water. By diluting the shampoo, you can avoid making too many suds that are hard to rinse out.

2 Spray head: Lift each braid and spray your head with the shampoo that has been watered down. To clean, gently rub your scalp with your fingers.

3. Rinse Well: Use lukewarm water to rinse your hair well. Be gentle so you don't mess up the braids.

4. Hair conditioner: Use a light conditioner on the length of your braids but don't put it on your head. Put it on for a while and then wash your face with cool water.

5. Pat Dry: Use a clean towel to pat your braids dry. Do not rub them, as this can make them frizzy.

<u>***Taking care of braided hair:***</u>

1. Leave-In Conditioner: To keep your braids wet, use a leave-in conditioner or braid spray every day.

2. Massage oil into your head every once in a while. Use a light hair oil or a natural oil like jojoba or argan oil. This keeps your hair from getting dry and itchy.

HOW TO REMOVE BRAIDS SAFELY AND CHANGE STYLES

To keep your natural hair from getting damaged, taking off braids can be a tricky process.

<u>***Here's the right way to do it***</u>

1. Get your tools ready. You'll need scissors, hair clips, and a comb or brush that can help you get rid of knots.

2. Cut the Ends Carefully: • Carefully cut off the ends of each braid where they are tied or held in place. Be careful not to cut your own hair.

3. Carefully unbraid: • Start at the bottom of each braid and slowly pull the ends apart. Take your time so that you don't twist or break the hair.

4. Detangle and condition: • Use a detangling comb or brush to gently detangle your normal hair after taking out all the extensions. Use a lot of conditioner to make the process go more smoothly.

5. Shampoo and condition: Use a shampoo without sulphates to wash your hair, and then condition it well. You can be sure that your natural hair is clean and moisturised after this.

6. Cut off any split ends: If you see any broken or split ends in your hair, you might want to cut them off to help your hair grow in a healthy way.

7. Styling to Protect: • Give your hair a break after taking out the braids before putting them back on. Choose styles that will keep you safe, like twists or low-manipulation styles.

<u>Keeping your hair safe while you sleep and do physical activities</u>

1. Tips for Sleeping: • Use a silk or satin cover to keep your hair from frizzing up.

• Before going to bed, you might want to wrap your hair in a silk or satin scarf or hat.

• If your braids are long, use a scrunchie or a cloth hair tie to tie them off lightly so they don't get tangled.

2. Physical Activities: • If you work out, you might want to wear a sweatband or headband to protect your sides and keep sweat from messing up your braids.

• When you work out, use a hair tie or scarf to keep your braids in a protective

way so they don't move around too much and cause friction.

Taking care of your braided hair is important for keeping it looking nice and for keeping your natural hair healthy. If you take good care of your hair, you can keep your braided style for a long time while keeping it healthy and vibrant. Cleaning your scalp, keeping it moist, and using low-manipulation methods on a regular basis will help your braids last longer and avoid damage. When it's time to take out your braids, be gentle, and be careful when switching to other types.

Q1: How often should you wash your braided hair and scalp? It depends on the type of hair you have and how active you are. Don't wash your hair too much, because it can lose its natural oils.

What kind of shampoo can I use on my braids?

A2: It's best to use a shampoo that doesn't have sulphates, but you can add water to regular shampoo to make it better for cleaning your scalp without making your braids too wet.

Q3: Are there certain items I shouldn't use on braided hair?

A3: Stay away from heavy, greasy products and those with alcohol because they can make your hair feel heavy and cause buildup. Choose natural oils and products that are light and made with water.

Q4: How can braids help a scalp that is itchy?

A4: To stop itching, use a shampoo for the scalp or dry shampoo in between washes. To soothe your scalp, you can also use a light hair oil or aloe vera gel.

Q5: If I braid my hair, can I swim?

A5: Yes, you can swim with braids on, but be careful. Before you go swimming, wet your hair with clean water to keep chlorine and saltwater from getting into your hair. After that, give your hair a good wash and condition.

Q6: What can I do to keep my braids from getting frizzy?

A6: Don't use too much friction or manipulation. Slip your long braids into a silk or satin pillowcase while you sleep, and use leave-in conditioner or braid spray to keep them moist.

Q7: How do I pick braids that are the right size and length?

A7: The length and size of your braids will depend on your hair type, style, and way of life. Talk to a professional braider to figure out what your best options are.

Q8: Can I use hair extensions from one set of braids on another?

A8: Yes, you can reuse hair extensions, but you must clean and sanitise them completely before putting them back on. Hair quality and cleanliness are very important things to think about.

Q9 Should I cut my natural hair after taking out the braids?

A9: To keep your hair healthy, trimming split ends is a good thing to do after taking out braids. That being said, you don't have to trim unless you see major damage.

Q10: How can I keep my edges safe while I have braids on?

A10: Styles that are too tight or heavy can hurt your edges. Don't use too many edge control products. Instead, protect your edges by putting oil or aloe vera gel on them.

Keep in mind that everyone has different hair and style preferences, so it's important to make these tips fit your needs. Giving your braided hair and natural hair regular care and attention will help them look great and stay healthy.

THE END